Keto For C_ 01

Lose Weight, Increase Energy and Stay Healthy with Amazing and Flavorful Recipes.

Lisa Flanary

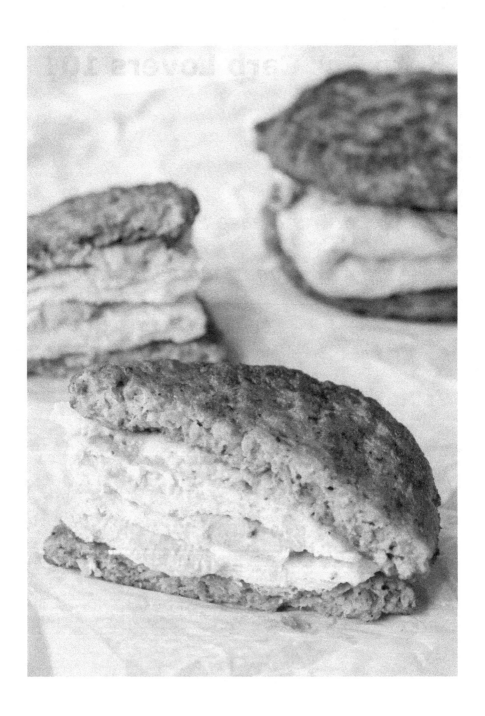

This declaration is deemed fair and valid by both the American Bar Association and the Committee of Publishers Association and is legally binding throughout the United States.

Furthermore, the transmission, duplication, or reproduction of any of the following work including specific information will be considered an illegal act irrespective of if it is done electronically or in print. This extends to creating a secondary or tertiary copy of the work or a recorded copy and is only allowed with the express written consent from the Publisher. All additional right reserved.

The information in the following pages is broadly considered a truthful and accurate account of facts and as such, any inattention, use, or misuse of the information in question by the reader will render any resulting actions solely under their purview. There are no scenarios in which the publisher or the original author of this work can be in any fashion deemed liable for any hardship or damages that may befall them after undertaking information described herein.

Additionally, the information in the following pages is intended only for informational purposes and should thus be thought of as universal. As befitting its nature, it is presented without assurance regarding its prolonged validity or interim quality. Trademarks that are mentioned are done without written consent and can in no way be considered an endorsement from the trademark holder.

Table of Contents

BREAKFAST

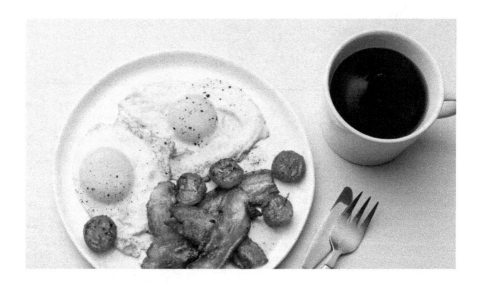

1. Crock Pot Keto

Preparation time: 15 minutes

Cooking time: 2 hours

Servings: 2

Ingredients:

- almond flour3 tablespoons

- coconut flour 1/2 tablespoon

- butter 1 tablespoon - egg 1 large

- sea salt1 pinch

- baking soda1/2 teaspoons

- salt

Directions:

1. Take a medium-sized skillet, melt the butter. It usually takes 20-30 seconds.

2. Pour coconut and almond flour, egg, salt into the melted butter and stir everything well.

3. Remove skillet from the heat and add baking soda.

4. Coat the slow cooker with cooking spray. Pour the mixture. Put on low for 2 hours. Check the readiness with a fork.

5. Remove the baked muffin from the slow cooker and eat with bacon slices, cheese, or other breakfast staples.

Nutrition: Calories: 321

Carbohydrate: 5 g

Protein: 23 g

Fat: 13.9 g

Sugar: 2.4 g

Sodium: 67 mg

Fiber: 11

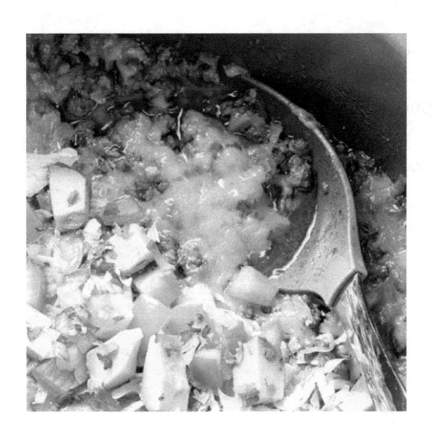

2.   Cauliflower Casserole with Tomato and Goat Cheese

Preparation time: 15 minutes

Cooking time: 3 hours

Servings: 2

Ingredients:

- cauliflower florets 6 cups
- olive oil 4 teaspoons
- dried oregano 1 teaspoon
- salt 1/2 teaspoon
- ground pepper 1/2 teaspoons
- Goat cheese crumbled 2 oz.
- The Sauce:
- olive oil 1 teaspoon

- garlic 3 cloves

- crushed tomatoes 1 (28 oz.) can

- bay leaves 2 pcs

- salt 1/4 teaspoon

- minced flat-leaf parsley 1/4 cup

Directions:

1. Grease the slow cooker with cooking spray, put the cauliflower on its bottom, and add olive oil, oregano, and pepper. Salt if desired.

2. Cook on the low setting within 2 hours until the cauliflower florets get tender and a little bit brown color.

3. For making the sauce: Take a medium-sized skillet, heat the olive oil, add garlic and cook 1 minute, stir it thoroughly all the time.

4. Add the crushed tomatoes and bay leaves; let it simmer for some minutes. Remove the bay leaves, dress with pepper and salt.

5. Put the sauce over the cauliflower florets in the slow cooker once the time is over.

6. Spread the Goat cheese over the dish, cover the slow cooker, and continue cooking for 1 hour on low. Serve warm!

Nutrition: Calories: 328

Carbohydrate: 3.5 g

Protein: 23 g Fat: 11 g

Sugar: 5 g

Sodium: 100 mg

Fiber: 13g

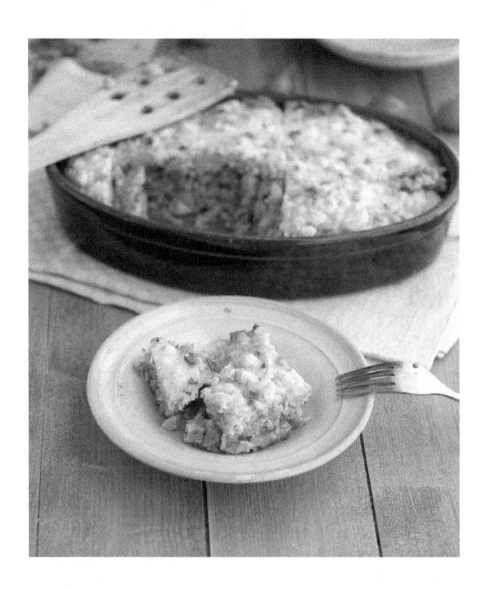

3. Greek Eggs Breakfast Casserole

Preparation time: 15 minutes

Cooking time: 6 hours

Servings: 2

Ingredients:

- eggs (whisked) 12 pcs
- milk 1/2 cup
- salt 1/2 teaspoon
- black pepper 1 teaspoon
- Red Onion 1 tablespoon
- Garlic 1 teaspoon
- Sun-dried tomatoes 1/2 cup
- spinach 2 cups
- Feta Cheese 1/2 cup crushed

- pepper at will

Directions:

1. Whisk the eggs in a bowl.

2. Add to the mixture milk, pepper, salt, and stir to combine. Add the minced onion and garlic.

3. Add dried tomatoes and spinach. Pour all the batter into the slow cooker, add Feta cheese. Set to cook on the low setting within 5-6 hours. Serve.

Nutrition: Calories: 365

Carbohydrate: 1.9 g

Protein: 23 g

Fat: 34 g

Sugar: 3.4 g

Sodium: 32 mg

Fiber: 11

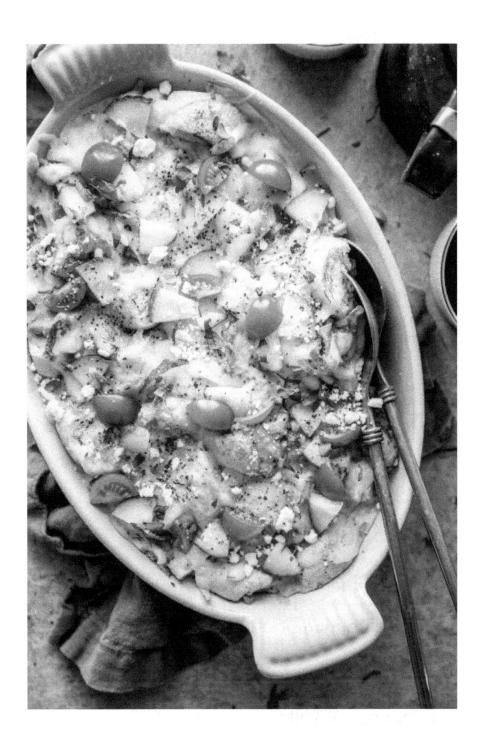

4. Crock Pot Turkish Breakfast Eggs

Preparation time: 15 minutes

Cooking time: 4 hours

Servings: 2

Ingredients:

- olive oil 1 tablespoon

- onions 2 pcs, chopped

- red bell pepper 1 pcs, sliced

- red chili 1 small - cherry tomatoes 8 pcs

- keto bread 1 slice

- eggs 4 pcs - milk 2 tablespoons

- small bunch of parsley, chopped

- natural yogurt 4 tablespoon

- pepper at will

Directions:

1. Grease the slow cooker using oil.

2. Heat-up, the oil, add the onions, pepper, and chili in a large skillet, then stir. Cook until the veggies begin to soften.

3. Transfer it in the Slow Cooker, then add the cherry tomatoes and bread, stir everything well.

4. Cook on low for 4 hours—season with fresh parsley and yogurt.

Nutrition: Calories: 123

Carbohydrate: 3.5 g

Protein: 32 g Fat: 19 g

Sugar: 3.4 g

Sodium: 100 mg

Fiber: 13g

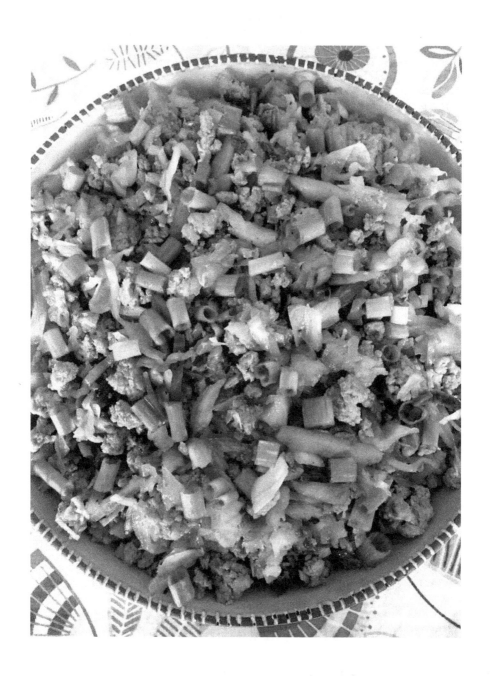

5.   Cheesy Garlic Brussels Sprouts

Preparation time: 15 minutes

Cooking time: 3 hours

Servings: 2

Ingredients:

- 1tablespoon unsalted butter
- 21/2 pounds Brussels sprouts, trimmed and halved
- 3/4 cup grated Parmesan cheese
- 2tablespoons heavy cream
- 1/8teaspoon freshly grated nutmeg
- 4cloves garlic, thinly sliced
- 4ounces cream cheese, cubed
- 1/2teaspoon kosher salt

- 1/4teaspoon ground black pepper

Directions:

1. Coat the insert of a 4- to – 6-quart crockpot with the butter. Add the garlic, cream cheese, Brussels sprouts, pepper, and salt.

2. Toss to mix very well—cover and cook on the low, about 2 to 3 hours.

3. Turn off the slow cooker. Stir in cream, parmesan, and nutmeg until the cheeses thaw and the Brussels sprouts are coated in a creamy sauce. Taste, season with more pepper if required. Serve.

Nutrition: Calories: 356

Carbohydrate: 1.0 g

Protein: 23 g

Fat: 34 g

Sugar: 3.4 g

Sodium: 56 mg

Fiber: 9

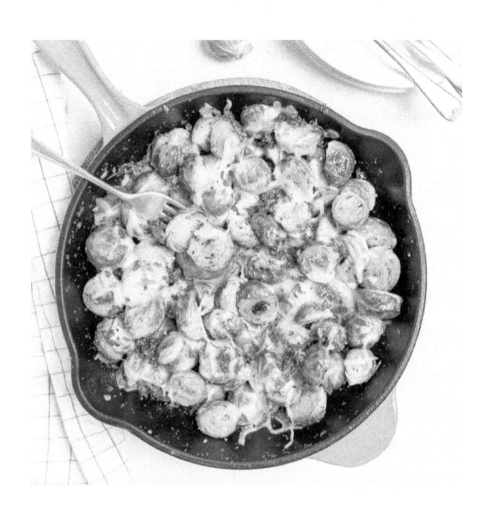

6.   Blueberry Pancake

Preparation time: 15 minutes

Cooking time: 40 minutes

Servings: 2

Ingredients:

- 11/2 cups milk

- 2large eggs

- 1teaspoon vanilla

- 2 cups all-purpose flour

- 21/2 teaspoon baking powder

- 2tablespoons white sugar

- 1/4cup fresh blueberries

Directions:

1. Toss the eggs, vanilla, and milk together in a small bowl. Stir flour, sugar, and baking powder together in a large bowl until well-mixed.

2. Add the wet fixings to the dry and stir just until mixed.

3. Pour the batter into the slow cooker. Add the blueberries.

4. Set the timer at 40 minutes on low.

5. Check to confirm if the pancake is cooked through by pressing the top. Serve and enjoy with syrup, fruit, or whipped cream.

Nutrition: Calories: 453 Carbohydrate: 2 g Protein: 56 g Fat: 76 g Sugar: 3 g Sodium: 65 mg Fiber: 11

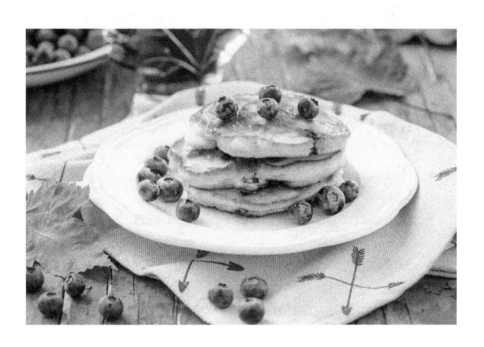

7.   Sausage and Peppers

Preparation time: 15 minutes

Cooking time: 6 hours

Servings: 2

Ingredients:

- 6 medium cloves garlic
- 2large yellow onions
- 4green bell peppers, cleaned and thinly sliced
- 28ounces canned unsalted crushed tomatoes
- 1/4cup of cold water - 1 bay leaf
- 2pounds uncooked Italian Sausage Links, mild or spicy

- 1tablespoon kosher salt

- 1teaspoon Italian seasoning

- 1/4teaspoon dried oregano

- 1/2teaspoon crushed red pepper flakes

Directions:

1. Thinly slice the garlic. Peel the onions and halve, then cut. Add the chopped garlic and sliced onion into the slow cooker. Remember to spray the slow cooker with oil. Cut the bell peppers in half.

2. Remove the ribs and any seeds in them. Then slice thinly.

3. Add the sliced bell peppers, Italian seasoning, salt, crushed red pepper flakes, dried oregano, 1 can crushed

tomatoes, and 1/4 cup of water to the slow cooker.

4. Toss to coat and liquid is uniformly distributed. Take out almost half of the peppers and the onion mixture to a bowl.

5. Immerse the uncooked sausage in the middle and then add the peppers and the onions back to the slow cooker.

6. Put the bay leaf, then cover, set to low, and cook for 6 hours. Serve hot.

Nutrition: Calories: 342

Carbohydrate: 1 g

Protein: 65 g

Fat: 28 g

Sugar: 4 g

Sodium: 67 mg

Fiber: 34 g

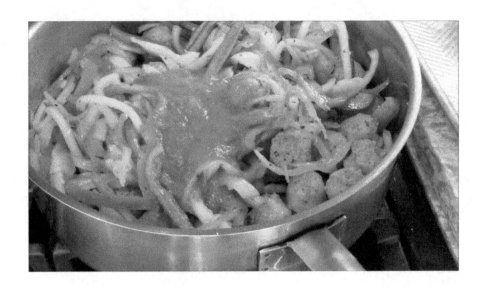

8. Breakfast Sausage Casserole

Preparation time: 15 minutes

Cooking time: 3 hours

Servings: 2

Ingredients:

- 1lb. pork sausage

- 1/2cup chopped green bell pepper

- 1/2cup chopped red bell pepper

- 1tablespoon ghee

- 12large eggs

- 1/2cup of coconut milk

- 1tablespoon nutritional yeast

- 1teaspoon dry rubbed sage

- 1teaspoon dried thyme

- 1/2teaspoon garlic powder

- 1/2teaspoon ground black pepper

- 1/2teaspoon salt

- 1/2cup sliced red onion

Directions:

1. Heat-up a medium cast-iron skillet over medium heat for 2 minutes. Add the pork sausage, then break it into small crumbles.

2. Cook for 3 minutes. Stir in the black pepper, sea salt, thyme, sage, and garlic powder.

3. Cook for an additional 5 minutes. Turn the heat off.

4. Stir in the bell peppers and the chopped onion. Coat the bowl of the slow cooker with ghee.

5. Add the pork and vegetable mixture into the bottom of the crockpot.

6. Whisk the coconut milk, nutritional yeast, and the eggs until the eggs are well incorporated together in a large bowl. Pour it into the crockpot on top of the pork mixture.

7. Cook on low for 2 to 3 hours. Chop into 6 servings.

Nutrition: Calories: 342

Carbohydrate: 1 g

Protein: 65 g

Fat: 28 g

Sugar: 4 g

Sodium: 67 mg

Fiber: 34 g

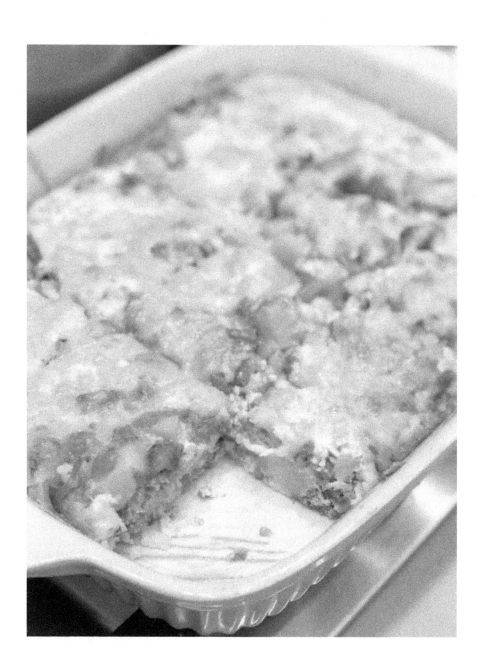

LUNCH

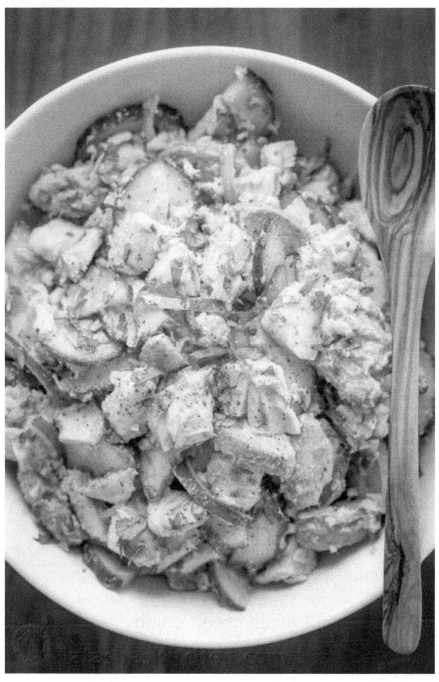

9.   Crockpot Chicken Adobo

Preparation time: 10 minutes

Cooking time: 8 hours

Servings: 2

Ingredients:

- 1/4cup of apple cider vinegar

- 12chicken drumsticks

- 1onion, diced into slices

- 2tablespoons of olive oil

- 10cloves garlic, smashed

- 1cup of gluten-free tamari

- 1/4cup of diced green onion

Directions:

1. Place the drumsticks in the Crockpot and then add the remaining Ingredients on top.

2. Cover it and cook for 8 hours on Low Settings.

3. Mix gently, then serve warm.

Nutrition: Calories 249

Fat 11.9 g

Carbs 1.8 g

Fiber 1.1 g

Sugar 0.3 g

Protein 25 g

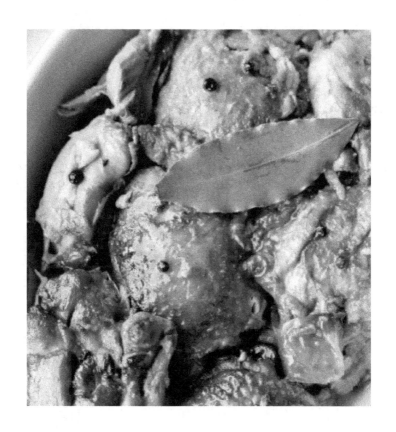

10. Chicken Ginger Curry

Preparation time: 10 minutes

Cooking time: 6 hours

Servings: 2

Ingredients:

- 11/2lb. chicken drumsticks (approx. 5 drumsticks), skin removed
- 1can coconut milk
- 1onion, diced
- 4 cloves garlic, minced
- 1-inch knob fresh ginger, minced
- 1Serrano pepper, minced
- 1tablespoon of Garam Masala
- 1/2teaspoon of cayenne

- 1/2teaspoon of paprika

- 1/2teaspoon of turmeric

- salt and pepper, adjust to taste

Directions:

1. Start by throwing all the Ingredients into the Crockpot.

2. Cover it and cook for 6 hours on Low Settings.

3. Garnish as desired.

4. Serve warm.

Nutrition:

Calories 248

Fat 15.7 g

Carbs 4 g

Fiber 0g

Sugar 1.1 g

Protein 14.1 g

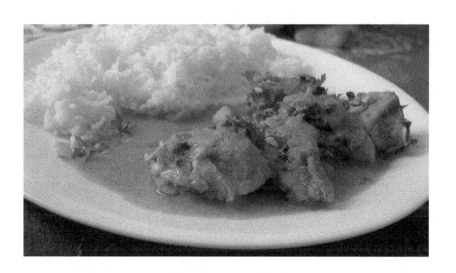

11. Thai Chicken Curry

Preparation time: 10 minutes

Cooking time: 2.5 hours

Servings: 2

Ingredients:

- 1can coconut milk

- 1/2cup of chicken stock

- 1lb. boneless, skinless chicken thighs, diced

- 12tablespoons of red curry paste

- 1tablespoon of coconut aminos

- 1tablespoon of fish sauce

- 2 3garlic cloves, minced

- Salt and black pepper-to taste

- red pepper flakes as desired

- 1bag frozen mixed veggies

Directions:

1. Start by throwing all the Ingredient except vegetables into the Crockpot.

2. Cover it and cook for 2 hours on Low Settings.

3. Remove its lid and thawed veggies.

4. Cover the crockpot again then continue cooking for another 30 minutes on Low settings.

5. Garnish as desired.

6. Serve warm.

Nutrition:

Calories 327

Fat 3.5 g

Carbs 4.6g

Fiber 0.4 g

Sugar 0.5 g

Protein 21.5 g

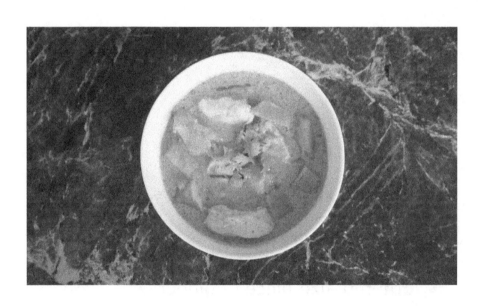

12. Lemongrass and Coconut Chicken Drumsticks

Preparation time: 10 minutes

Cooking time: 5 hours

Servings: 2

Ingredients:

- 10drumsticks, skin removed

- 1thick stalk fresh lemongrass

- 4cloves garlic, minced

- 1thumb-size piece of ginger

- 1cup of coconut milk

- 2tablespoons of Red Boat fish sauce

- 3tablespoons of coconut aminos

- 1teaspoon of five-spice powder

- 1large onion, sliced

- 1/4cup of fresh scallions, diced

- Kosher salt

- Black pepper

Directions:

1. Start by throwing all the Ingredient into the Crockpot.

2. Cover it and cook for 5 hours on Low Settings.

3. Garnish as desired.

4. Serve warm.

Nutrition:

Calories 372

Fat 11.1 g

Carbs 0.9 g

Fiber 0.2 g

Sugar 0.2 g

Protein 63.5 g

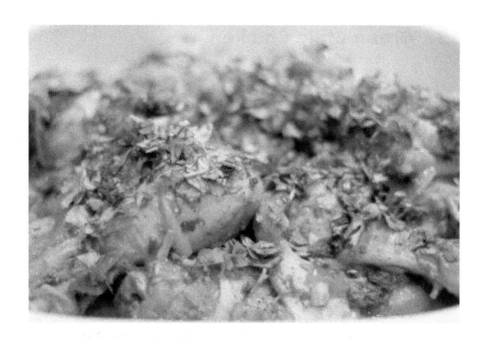

13. Green Chile Chicken

Preparation time: 10 minutes

Cooking time: 6 hours

Servings: 2

Ingredients:

- 8chicken thighs, thawed, boneless and skinless
- 1can green chilies
- 2teaspoons of garlic salt
- optional: add in 1/2 cup of diced onions

Directions:

1. Start by throwing all the Ingredients into the Crockpot.

2. Cover it and cook for 6 hours on Low Settings.

3. Garnish as desired.

4. Serve warm.

Nutrition: Calories 248 Fat 2.4 g Carbs 2.9 g Fiber 0.7 g Sugar 0.7 g Protein 44.3 g

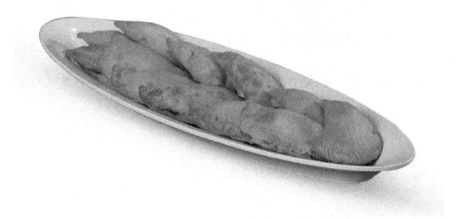

14. Garlic Butter Chicken with Cream Cheese Sauce

Preparation time: 10 minutes

Cooking time: 6 hours

Servings: 2

Ingredients:

For the garlic chicken:

- 8garlic cloves, sliced

- 1.5teaspoons of salt

- 1stick of butter

- 2 2.5lb. of chicken breasts

- Optional 1 onion, sliced

For the cream cheese sauce:

- 8oz. of cream cheese

- 1cup of chicken stock

- salt to taste

Directions:

1. Start by throwing all the Ingredients for garlic chicken into the Crockpot.

2. Cover it and cook for 6 hours on Low Settings.

3. Now stir cook all the Ingredients for cream cheese sauce in a saucepan.

4. Once heated, pour this sauce over the cooked chicken.

5. Garnish as desired.

6. Serve warm.

Nutrition: Calories 301 Fat 12.2 g Carbs 1.5 g

Fiber 0.9 g Sugar 1.4 g Protein 28.8 g

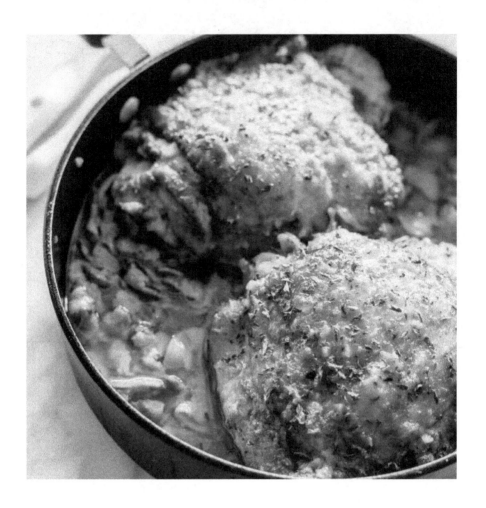

15. Spicy Wings with Mint Sauce

Preparation time: 10 minutes

Cooking time: 6 hours

Servings: 2

Ingredients:

- 1tablespoon of cumin

- 18chicken wings, cut in half

- 1tablespoon of turmeric

- 1tablespoon of coriander

- 1tablespoon of fresh ginger, finely grated

- 2tablespoon of olive oil

- tablespoon of paprika

- A pinch of cayenne pepper

- 1/4cup of chicken stock

- Salt and black pepper ground, to taste

- Chutney/ Sauce:

- 1cup of fresh mint leaves

- Juice of 1/2 lime

- 3/4cup of cilantro

- 1Serrano pepper

- 1tablespoon of water

- 1small ginger piece, peeled and diced

- 1tablespoon of olive oil

- Salt and black pepper ground, to taste

Directions:

1. Start by throwing all the Ingredients for wings into the Crockpot.

2. Cover it and cook for 6 hours on Low Settings.

3. Meanwhile, blend all the mint sauce Ingredients in a blender jug.

4. Serve the cooked wings with mint sauce.

5. Garnish as desired.

6. Serve warm.

Nutrition: Calories 248 Fat 15.7 g Total Carbs 0.4 g Fiber 0g Sugar 0 g Protein 24.9 g

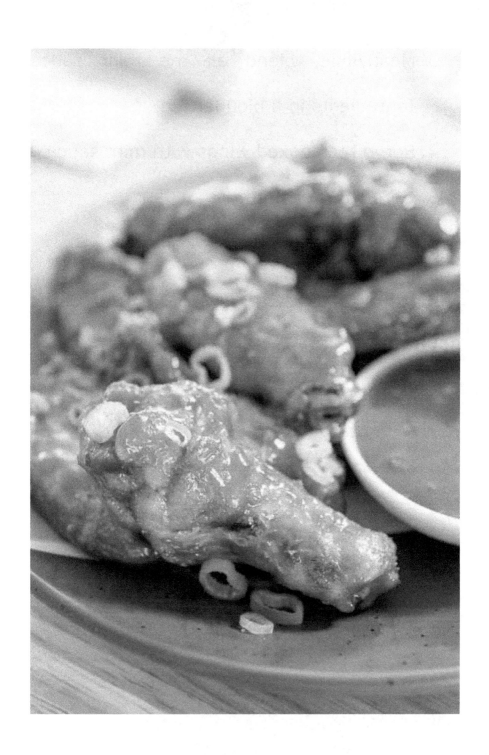

16. Marinara-Braised Turkey Meatballs

Preparation time: 15 minutes

Cooking time: 6 hours

Servings: 2

Ingredients:

- 3Tablespoons Extra-Virgin Olive Oil

- 1Pound Ground Turkey

- 1Pound Breakfast Sausage

- 1/2Cup Almond Flour

- 1Egg

- 1Tablespoon Chopped Basil

- 2Teaspoons Chopped Oregano

- 1/2Teaspoon Salt

- 1/4Teaspoon Freshly Ground Black Pepper

- 2Cups Simple Marinara Sauce

- 1Cup Shredded Mozzarella Cheese

Directions:

1. Lightly grease the insert of the slow cooker with 1 tablespoon of the olive oil.

2. In a large bowl, mix together the turkey, sausage, almond flour, egg, basil, oregano, salt, and pepper. Roll the mixture into golf ball–sized meatballs.

3. In a large skillet over medium-high heat, heat the remaining 2 tablespoons of the olive oil. Add the meatballs and brown for 7 minutes, turning several times.

4. Transfer the meatballs to the insert and add the marinara sauce.

5. Cover and cook on low for 6 hours.

6. Serve topped with the mozzarella cheese.

Nutrition: Calories 248 Fat 15.7 g Total Carbs 0.4 g Fiber 0g Sugar 0 g Protein 24.9 g

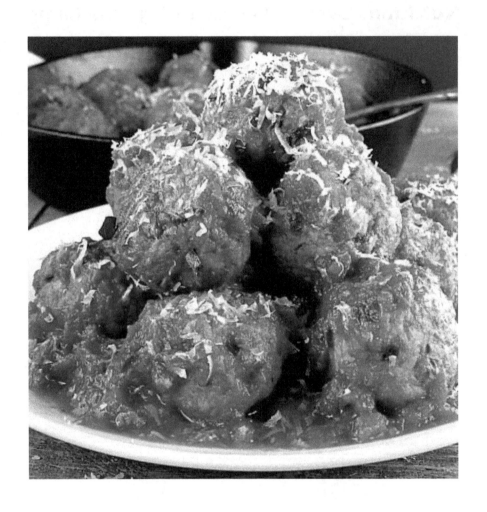

DINNER

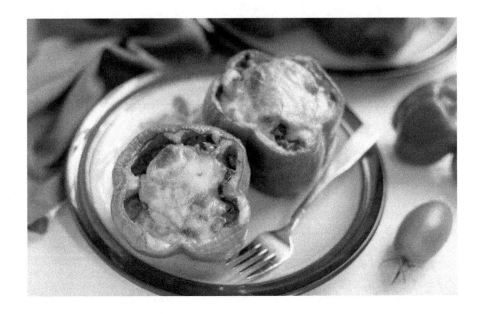

17. Shrimp Curry

Preparation Time: 15 minutes

Cooking time: 2 hrs.

Servings: 2

Ingredients

- 1-pound shrimp, peeled and deveined

- 1 tablespoon red curry paste

- 1 teaspoon curry powder

- 1 cup of coconut milk

- 1 tablespoon curry paste

- 1/3 jalapeno pepper, chopped

- 1/2 teaspoon garlic powder

- 1 teaspoon olive oil

- 1/2 cup spring onions, chopped

Directions:

1. In the slow cooker, mix the shrimp with curry paste and the other ingredients.
2. Close the lid and cook the curry for 1.5 hours on High.

Nutrition:

Calories 261

Fat 13.8

Fiber 1.7

Carbs 5,

Protein 21

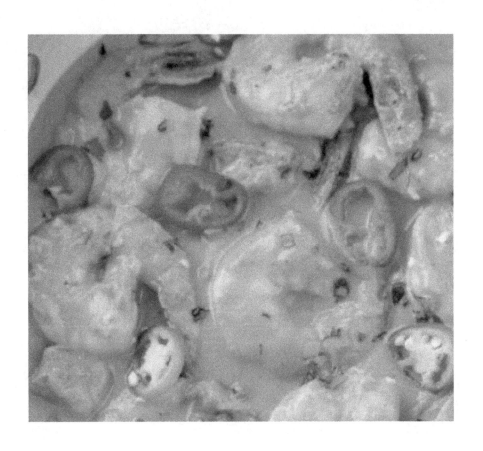

18. Salmon with Leeks and Cream

Preparation Time: 15 minutes

Cooking time: 4 hrs.

Servings: 2

Ingredients

- 4 fresh salmon fillets

- One leek, finely sliced

- 1 cup heavy cream

- 1/2 cup white wine

Directions:

1. Pour the cream and wine into a pot, bring to a simmer and reduce until slightly thickened.

2. Rub the salmon fillets with olive oil, and sprinkle with salt and pepper.

3. Drizzle some olive oil into the Slow Cooker.

4. Add the leeks to the pot and sprinkle with salt and pepper.

5. Place the salmon fillets on top of the leeks.

6. Pour the reduced cream and wine mixture into the pot.

7. Place the lid onto the pot and set the temperature to LOW.

8. Cook for 4 hours.

9. Serve the salmon with a generous serving of leeks and creamy sauce!

Nutrition: Calories 132

Fat 12.8

Fiber 1

Carbs 4,

Protein 15

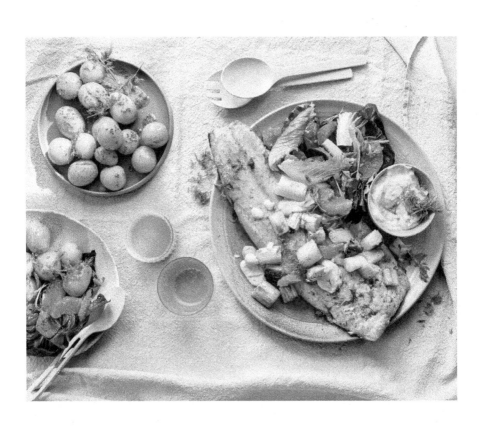

19. Shrimp Tomato Medley

Preparation Time: 15 minutes

Cooking time: 4 hrs.

Servings: 2

Ingredients

- 4 scallions, diced

- 11/2 tablespoon of coconut oil

- 1 small ginger root, diced

- 8 cups of chicken stock

- 1/4 cup of coconut amino

- 1/4 teaspoon of fish sauce

- 1 lb. shrimp, peeled and deveined

- 1/2 lb. tomatoes

- Black pepper ground, to taste

- 1 tablespoon of sesame oil

- 1 (5 oz.) can bamboo shoots, sliced

Directions:

1. Start by throwing all the Ingredients: into your Crockpot.

2. Cover its lid and cook for 1 hour on Low setting.

3. Once done, remove its lid and give it a stir.

4. Serve warm.

Nutrition:

Calories 371

Fat 3.7 g

Sodium 121 mg

Carbs 4 g

Fiber 1.5 g

Protein 26.5 g

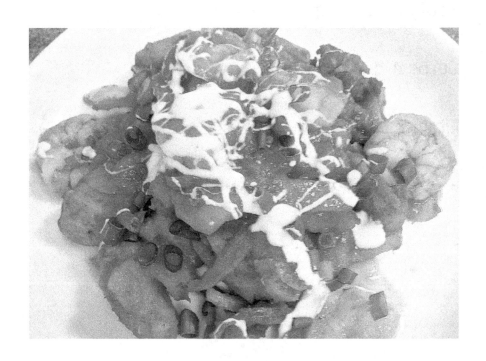

20. Fish and Tomato Stew

Preparation Time: 15 minutes

Cooking time: 4 hrs.

Servings: 2

Ingredients

- 4 tomatoes, chopped

- 2 cups fish stock

- 5 garlic cloves, finely chopped

- 1 tsp. ground cumin

- 1 tsp. ground chili

- 1 tsp. ground coriander

- 3 large white fish fillets, cut into chunks

- Handful of fresh parsley, chopped

Directions:

1. Drizzle some olive oil into the Slow Cooker.

2. Add the tinned tomatoes, fish stock, garlic, cumin, chili, coriander, fish, salt, and pepper, stir to combine.

3. Place the lid onto the pot and set the temperature to HIGH.

4. Cook for 4 hours.

5. Serve the stew while hot, with a generous sprinkling of fresh parsley!

Nutrition: Calories 326771

Fat 3.7 g Sodium

121 mg Carbs

3 g Fiber 2 g

Protein 28 g

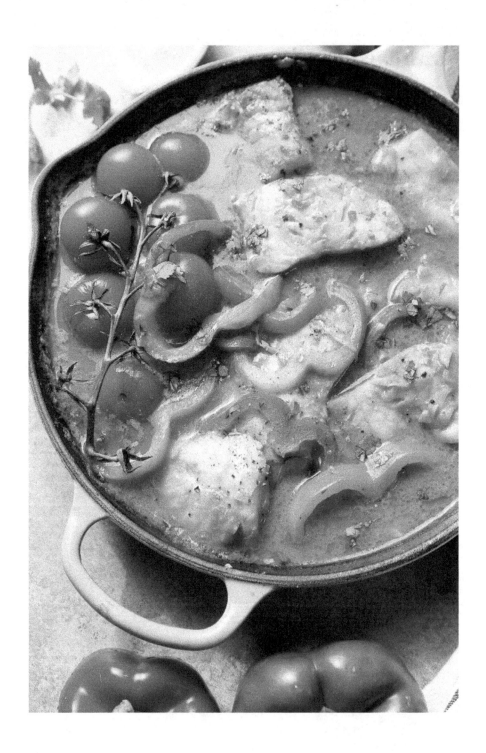

21. Shrimp And Zucchini

Preparation Time: 6 minutes

Cooking time: 4 hrs.

Servings: 2

Ingredients

- 1-pound shrimp, peeled and deveined

- 2 zucchinis, roughly cubed

- 1 cup cherry tomatoes, halved

- 1/2 cup Mozzarella cheese, shredded

- 4 tablespoons cream cheese

- 1 tablespoon butter, melted

- 1 teaspoon salt

- 1 tablespoon keto tomato sauce

- 3/4 cup of water

Directions:

1. In the slow cooker, mix the shrimp with zucchinis and the other ingredients except the cheese and toss.

2. Sprinkle the cheese on top, close the lid and cook on High for 2 hours.

Nutrition Calories 223 Fat 8.9 Fiber 0.8 Carbs 3.2 Protein 19.3

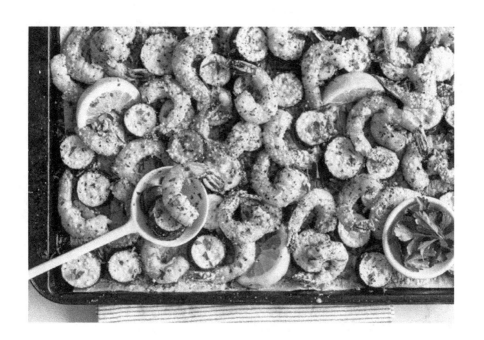

22. Coffee Creams with Toasted Seed Crumble Topping

Preparation Time: 6 minutes

Cooking time: 4 hrs.

Servings: 2

Ingredients

- 2 cups heavy cream

- 3 egg yolks, lightly beaten

- 1 tsp. vanilla extract

- 3 tbsp. strong espresso coffee (or 3tsp instant coffee dissolved in 3tbsp. boiling water)

- 1/2 cup mixed seeds – sesame seeds, pumpkin seeds, chia seeds, sunflower seeds,
- 1 tsp. cinnamon
- 1 tbsp. coconut oil

Directions:

1. Heat the coconut oil in a small fry pan until melted.

2. Add the mixed seeds, cinnamon, and a pinch of salt, toss in the oil and heat until toasted and golden, place into a small bowl and set aside.

3. In a medium-sized bowl, whisk together the cream, egg yolks, vanilla, and coffee.

4. Pour the cream/coffee mixture into the ramekins.

5. Place the ramekins into the Slow Cooker.

6. Pour enough hot water into the pot to reach half way up the ramekins.

7. Place the lid onto the pot and set the temperature to LOW.

8. Cook for 4 hours.

9. Remove the ramekins from the Slow Cooker and leave to cool slightly on the bench.

10.　　Sprinkle the seed mixture over the top of each custard before serving.

Nutrition

Calories 176

Fat 5

Fiber 1

Carbs 3

Protein 21

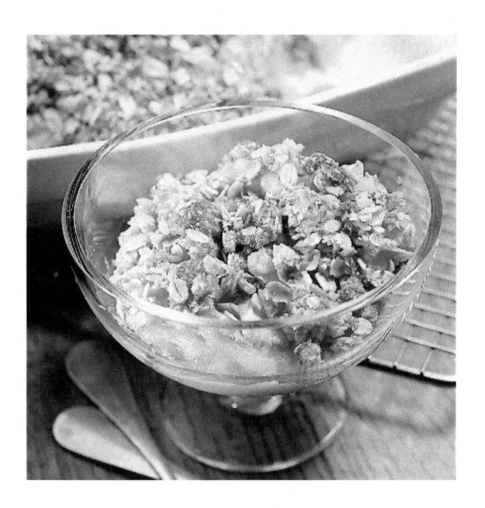

23. Cod & Peas with Sour Cream

Preparation Time: 6 minutes

Cooking time: 1 hrs.

Servings: 2

Ingredients

- 1 tablespoon of fresh parsley

- 1 garlic clove, diced

- 1/2 lb. frozen peas

- 1/2 teaspoon of paprika

- 1 cup of sour cream

- 1/2 cup of white wine

Directions:

1. Start by throwing all the Ingredients: into your Crockpot except sour cream.

2. Cover its lid and cook for 1 hour on High setting.

3. Once done, remove its lid and give it a stir.

4. Stir in sour cream and mix it gently

5. Serve warm.

Nutrition: Calories 349

Fat 31.9 g

Sodium 237 mg

Carbs 1.6 g

Sugar 1.4 g

Fiber 3.4 g

Protein 11 g

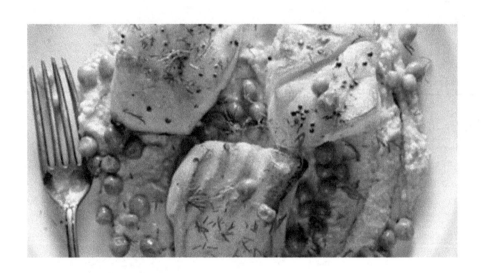

24. Slow Cooker Tuna Steaks

Preparation Time: 6 minutes

Cooking time: 4 hrs.

Servings: 2

Ingredients

- 4 tuna steaks

- 3 garlic cloves, crushed

- 1 lemon, sliced into 8 slices

- 1/2 cup white wine

Directions:

1. Reduce the white wine in a pot by simmering until the strong alcoholic smell is cooked off.

2. Rub the tuna steaks with olive oil, and sprinkle with salt and pepper.

3. Place the tuna steaks into the Slow Cooker.

4. Sprinkle the crushed garlic on top of the tuna steaks.

5. Place 2 lemon slices on top of each tuna steak.

6. Pour the reduced wine into the pot.

7. Secure the lid onto the pot and set the temperature to HIGH.

8. Cook for 3 hours.

9. Serve with a drizzle of leftover liquid from the pot, and a side of crispy greens!

Nutrition:

Calories 123

Fat 21 g

Sodium 213 mg

Carbs 2 g

Sugar 2 g

Fiber 3g

Protein 15 g

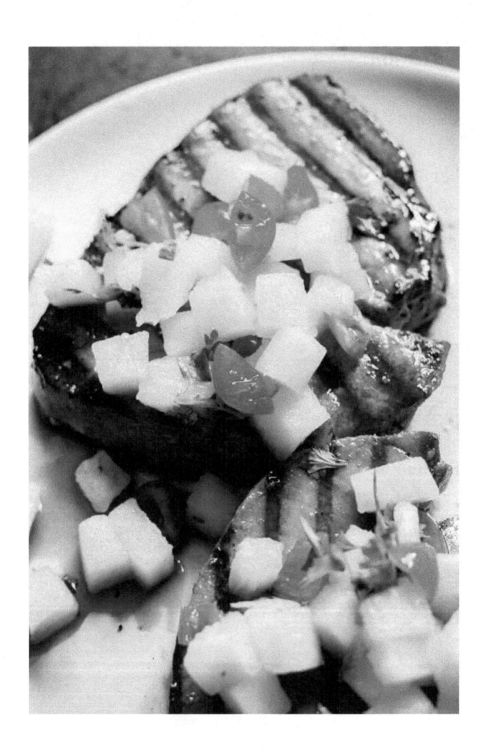

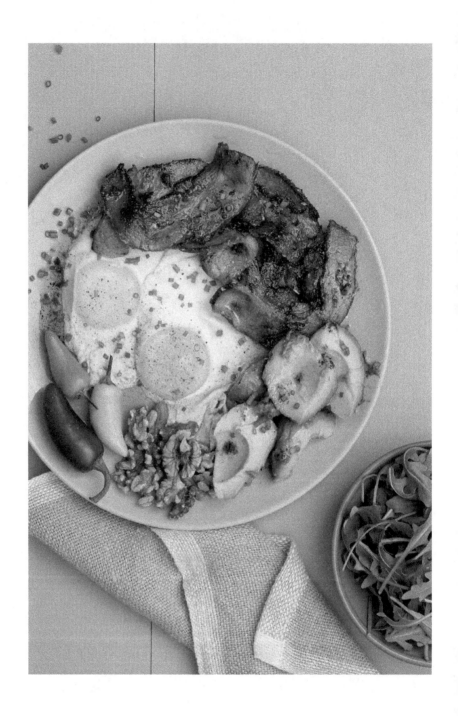

CPSIA information can be obtained
at www.ICGtesting.com
Printed in the USA
BVHW090547090621
609011BV00011B/2402

9 781803 040196